YOUR KNOWLEDGE HAS VALUE

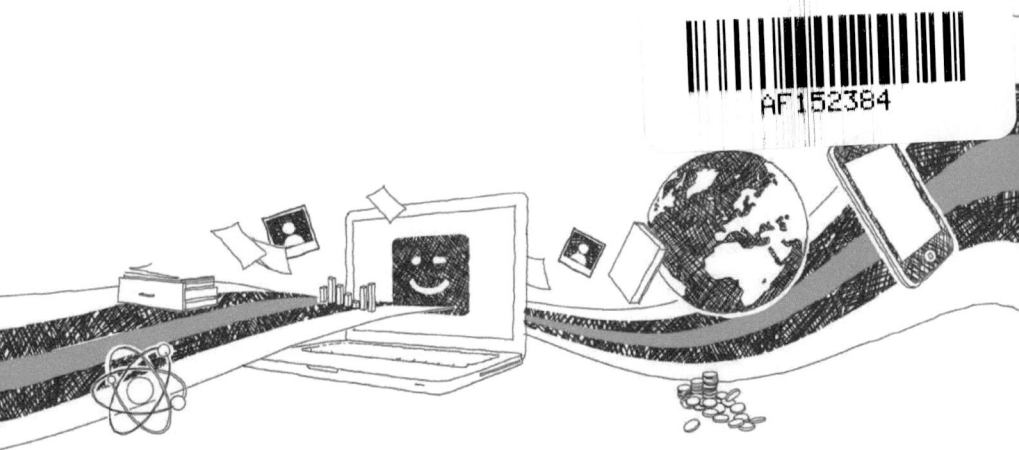
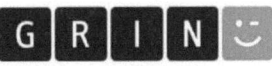

Dr. Peter Ubah Okeke

Vaginal Candidiasis and trichomoniasis infections in Pregnancy

Medical Microbiology

GRIN Publishing

Bibliographic information published by the German National Library:

The German National Library lists this publication in the National Bibliography; detailed bibliographic data are available on the Internet at http://dnb.dnb.de .

Imprint:

Copyright © 2013 GRIN Verlag GmbH
Print and binding: Books on Demand GmbH, Norderstedt Germany
ISBN: 978-3-656-48163-8

This book at GRIN:

http://www.grin.com/en/e-book/231669/vaginal-candidiasis-and-trichomoniasis-infections-in-pregnancy

GRIN - Your knowledge has value

Since its foundation in 1998, GRIN has specialized in publishing academic texts by students, college teachers and other academics as e-book and printed book. The website www.grin.com is an ideal platform for presenting term papers, final papers, scientific essays, dissertations and specialist books.

Visit us on the internet:

http://www.grin.com/

http://www.facebook.com/grincom

http://www.twitter.com/grin_com

Vaginal Candidiasis and trichomoniasis infections in pregnant women.

By

Dr. Peter Ubah Okeke

August, 2013

Research contents

Abstract

A hundred and twenty-seven (127) pregnant women performed high vaginal swab (HVS) tests between the months of May to July, 2013, the age range of the pregnant women studied were from 13 to 45 years old. The specimen were studied for candida species and trichomonas vaginalis infections using wet mount or direct examination with 10% Potassium hydroxide (KOH) added, and gram stain techniques. They results of 21.26 % was obtained for candida species, while 6.3% was infected with trichomonas vaginalis. The study observed that the infection rate of candida species among the pregnant women was statistically significant to that of trichomonas vaginalis, considering $P \leq 0.05$. The co-infection rate of the study was 0.79%. The infection of candida species of 28.8% was observed among primigravidae, while trichomonas vaginalis was 10.17%, the multigravidae registered 14.71% of candida species infection and trichomonas vaginalis was 2.94%. Therefore, the primigravidae were more infected with candida species and trichomonas vaginalis than multigravidae. The age groups of 13 to 25 years of the pregnant women were mostly infected by candida species (25.93%) and trichomonas vaginalis infection was 7.41%. The pregnant mothers at third trimester (27 to 40 weeks) were mostly attacked, making a prevalence rate of 23.81% of candida species, while trichomonas vaginalis was 9.52%.

The conclusion was that contributing factors such as douching should be avoided; indiscriminate use of antibiotics without medical supervision, and education of the pregnant women using various forms, stressing the importance of prevention and control strategies should be implemented.

Keywords: Vaginal candidiasis, Trichomoniasis, Pregnant, Women, Cape Verde.

Objective: To determine the frequency of candidiasis and trichomoniasis infections in pregnant women.

Limitations: The techniques of latex agglutination, Enzyme linked immunosorbent assay (ELISA), and cultural tests were not used in this work.

Introduction and literature review

Infections of the vulva and vagina are common among women and the most common types of vulvovaginitis are Candidiasis, trichomoniasis and bacterial vaginosis.

Candida species may be transmitted by sexual partners and may cause balanitis, balanoposthitis and rarely urethritis in men. However, for candida species to colonize the vagina, they must first adhere to the vaginal epithelial cells and then grow, proliferate, and germinate, before causing symptomatic inflammation. Changes in the vaginal environment are usually necessary before the organism can induce virulent pathological effects.

The natural bacterial flora serves as the most important defense mechanism against colonization and inflammation. The mechanism whereby candida species induces inflammation is not yet known, but essential predisposing factors for colonization and inflammation were; changes in reproductive hormone levels associated with premenstrual periods, pregnancy, oral contraceptive pills, abusive use of antibiotics and diabetes mellitus.

Chemical products, local allergy and delayed hypersensitivity can contribute to the induction of symptomatic vaginitis and vulvitis and may play a role in chronic or recurrent Candidiasis. The diagnosis of vaginal Candidiasis cannot always be confirmed on the basis of clinical symptoms alone without adequate laboratory investigations. Although, clinical suggestive diagnosis of Candidiasis includes; vaginal itching, an odorless curdy white discharge, burning sensation in the vulva region, dysuria and erythema of the labia and vulva, arriving at this, a consulting physician must rely dynamically and effectively on laboratory findings to confirm the diagnosis.

Candidiasis, an opportunistic infection is mainly caused by candida albicans, is one of the most common causes of vaginitis, Eschenbach D.A. (2004). Omar AA (2001) reported that the incidence of Candidiasis has increased markedly during the last three decades. The incidence of Candidiasis continued to double unabated in the third trimester of pregnancy and multigravida suffer significantly more than primigravida, Limia,O. F (2004). However, a significant proportion of women with chronic or recurrent Candidiasis first present with this infection while pregnant. The systems by which pregnancy encourages candida colonization are still very complex, Xu, DJ &Sobel JD (2004).

During pregnancy, levels of both progesterone and estrogen hormones are high. Progesterone has suppressive effects on the anti-candida activity of the neutrophils, Nohmi (1995), while estrogen is responsible for reducing the ability of vaginal epithelial cells to inhibit the growth of candida species and also decreases immunoglobulin in the vaginal exudates resulting in increased propensity of pregnant women to vaginal Candidiasis, Fidel (2005). It is a common gynaecologic problem that affects three out of four women in their lifetime, Das-Neves et al (2008).

Dr. Ferrer (2000) reported that more than 40% of affected women would have two or more cases of Candidiasis, with the vagina discharging smelly, thick, whitish-yellowish, itching, burning and swelling feelings presenting even in the healthiest of women. Akinbiyi et al (2008) stressed that candida vaginitis identification as a cause of disease can be a difficult task since almost 50% of asymptomatic women do have candida organisms as part of their endogenous vaginal flora, hence

4

limitations in using clinical signs and symptoms in the diagnosis of vaginal infection. Under normal condition, candida yeast is held in check by normal body defense mechanisms together with other normal microbial flora of the body. For example, the activity of the vagina is maintained at PH 4.0 – 4.5. This acidity level prevents some vaginal microbial flora from establishing as infection. The physiological changes in the balance of the body system would affect both beneficial and harmful yeasts, bacteria and other microorganisms in the body. This would in effect alter the acidic condition of the vagina reducing it to PH 5.0 – 6.5, and this gives room for the multiplication of microorganisms such as candida, Akinbiyi et al (2008). The PH of the vagina may increase with advancing age, phase of menstrual cycle, sexual activity, birth control pills, pregnancy, presence of necrotic or apoptotic tissue or foreign bodies and use of hygienic products or antibiotics, Nyirjesy (2008).

Candidiasis infection in pregnancy does not usually harm the unborn baby, but causes great discomfort to the mother, and if untreated, the baby can get infected (oral thrush) at birth, which poses a serious health problem in premature infants. However, untreated vaginal infection can cause pelvic inflammatory disease, a condition which can scar the fallopian tube and cause infertility in women, Garcia et al (2006).

Trichomoniasis on the other hand, is an infection of the genital tract caused by a flagellated protozoon, trichomonas vaginalis. Trichomoniasis is considered mainly as sexually transmitted, non-veneral transmission is not well documented or published. Vaginal trichomoniasis may be asymptomatic in a large proportion of infected women. In women therefore, trichomoniasis elicits an acute inflammatory response resulting in vaginal discharge containing high, moderate or low numbers of polymorphonuclear neutrophils. Typical symptoms associated with trichomoniasis in women include vaginal itching or irritation and a frothy grey to green- yellow discharge, vaginal malodor and dysuria.

Trichomonas vaginalis is an ovoid, globular pear shaped flagellate, 12 to 25 μm long, with four free anterior flagella and one extra posterior flagellum attached to an undulating membrane, extending along the length of its body. However, certain signs and symptoms are predictive for trichomoniasis, the detection of the parasite is necessary to establish the diagnosis. Trichomonads are best recognized by an experienced medical laboratory scientist or technician, by their typical jerky motility in a suspended wet preparation.

The parasite is passed from an infected sexual partner to an uninfected partner during sexual intercourse. During sexual intercourse, the parasite is usually transmitted from the penis to the vagina or from vagina to penis depending on who is infected. It can also pass from vagina to another vagina. However, it is not relatively common for the parasite to infect other body parts like, the hands, mouth, and anus. It is not clear why some patients with the infection get symptoms, while others are not, but it can probably depends on factors like the person's age and overall health condition. Although, infected people without symptoms can still pass the trichomonas vaginalis to others. Trichomoniasis can make one feel unpleasant during sex and without treatment; the infection can last for months or even years.

Despite a relative paucity of studies on the prevalence and incidence of trichomoniasis, the studies of Dr. Cates W. Jr. (1999), expressed that, trichomonas infection is one of the most common sexually transmitted diseases in the United States, with an estimated 5 million new cases each year. Although the microorganism appears to be highly prevalent and has a global geographic distribution, trichomonas has not been the focus of intensive research nor of active control programs.

Trichomoniasis is the most prevalent, non- viral, sexually transmitted infection worldwide, Shira & Frank (2006).In the United States, an estimated 3.7 million people have trichomonas vaginalis and only about 30% develop pathological signs of trichomoniasis. Infection rate is common in women than men and this risk increases with age. Although, the infection is associated with vaginitis and urethritis, the disease encircles a broad spectrum of symptoms, ranging from a severe inflammation and irritation with fruity malodorous discharge to a relatively asymptomatic carrier state. The World Health Organization estimates that 10% to 25% of vaginal infections is due to trichomoniasis, WHO (2001).

Trichomoniasis infection typically elicits an aggressive local cellular immune response with inflammation of the vaginal epithelium and exocervix in women, and the urethra of men, Sardana S. et al (1994). Trichomoniasis infection can increase the risk of transmission of Human immunodeficiency Virus (HIV), Cohen (2000). This inflammatory response induces a large infiltration of leucocytes, including HIV target cells such as CD4+ bearing T- lymphocytes and macrophages to which HIV can bind and gain access, Levine W.C et al (1998). In HIV negative person, both the leucocytes infiltration and genital lesions induced by trichomonas vaginalis may enlarge the portal of entry for HIV, by increasing the number of target cells for the virus and allowing direct viral access to the bloodstream through open lesions. Laconically, in HIV infected person, the hemorrhage and inflammation can increase the level of virus laden body fluids, the numbers of HIV infected lymphocytes and macrophages present in the genital contact area or both.

The resulting increase of both free virus and virus infected lymphocytes can expand the portal of exit, thereby increasing the chances of HIV exposure and transmission to an uninfected person. Increased cervical shedding of HIV has been shown to be associated with cervical inflammation, Kreiss, J et al (1994). Hobbs, M M et al (1999) documented substantial increased urethral viral loads in men with Trichomoniasis infection, in addition, trichomonas has the capacity to degrade secretory leukocyte protease inhibitor, a product known to block HIV cell attachment; this process may also promote HIV transmission, Draper, D et al (1998).

The cross-sectional study of Ghys P D et al (1995) among female sex workers in Abidjan, Ivory Coast, discovered an association between HIV and trichomonas infection in bivariate analysis, and the work of Ter Muelen J et al (1992) in Tanzania concluded that trichomonas infection was more common in women with HIV infection in multivariate analysis. However, these cross. Sectional studies are limited by the issue of temporal ambiguity, that is, lack of proper information on whether trichomonas infection preceded HIV. The evaluation of four hundred and thirty-one HIV negative women in Zaire by Laga M and co-workers stated that prior trichomonas infection was associated with a two fold increase rate of HIV seroconversion in a multivariate setting.

Sutton M et al (2007) reported the prevalence of Trichomonas vaginalis among women in the United States of America (USA) at 3.1% and proved that significant racial disparity exists in the USA, with black women tendency for infection with trichomonas been ten times higher than other races in the USA. This Phenomenon may indicate a high prevalence of trichomonas infection among the sex partners of these women. The association with black race in the USA may also reflect decreased use of barrier protection in this population. Alternatively, it is possible that practices such as douching, which is reportedly more common in black women, Aral S O et al (1992), and can increase susceptibility to other sexually transmission infections, Scholes D et al (1998), which in turn predispose to trichomoniasis and hence, explain the observed discrepancy racial association.

However, increased prevalence of trichomonas infection can also reflect lack of access to care and distrust of the health care system, which can manifest as failure to seek care, non-compliance with treatment recommendations, and also hesitation to refer partners for adequate treatment, drug use and its association with high risk sexual behaviors, including, but not exclusive to, trading sex for money or drugs, could also explain the racial disparity in the USA. Furthermore, compared with other racial ethnicities in the USA, a greater proportion of blacks are unmarried, divorced or legally separated, Bennett C (1993), and unmarried status is itself a risk marker for sexually transmission infections, Aral & Holmes (1989). Finally, the observed racial disparity can reflect strain differences of trichomonas, for example; if the strains that infect Afro-Americana are more likely to produce chronic, persistent infection of longer duration, higher prevalence would be observed, this scientific hypothesis has not yet been proved, again in this aspect further research is imperative.

By producing a wide array of glycosidase and cysteine proteinase enzymes, trichomonas vaginalis can easily adapt to the environment, harvesting host proteins and Deoxyribonucleic acid (DNA) for metabolism. With the propensity to cause lesions, vaginitis and acute inflammatory disease of the genital mucosa, trichomonas parasite acts as a potential catalyst in the acquisition of secondary infections including Human immunodeficiency virus (HIV) and human papillomavirus (HPV)- the organism responsible for the pathogenesis of cervical cancer, Rughooputh & Greenwell (2005).

Trichomoniasis infected pregnant mother stands the risk of adverse birth outcomes such as premature rupture of membrane, premature labour, low birth weight, and post abortion or post hysterectomy infection as well as infertility, and enhanced predisposition to neoplastic transformation in cervical tissues stated, Uneke et al (2006).

Methodology

Study area
This work was conducted in the city of Porto Novo, Santo Antâo, Cape Verde and the vaginal samples were tested at the department of Medical Laboratory Science section, Central Hospital, Porto Novo.

Period of the research
The collection of the vaginal samples and testing, for the purpose of this study started on First day of May, 2013 to thirty first of July, 2013 respectively.

Choice of patients
All pregnant women attending antenatal clinic for the first time in all the regions of Porto Novo were chosen for this work, and the trimesters, age, and parity of the pregnant women were recorded.

Collection of specimens

A Total of one hundred and twenty –seven (127) pregnant women were selected and vaginal discharge was removed from the vaginal walls of the pregnant women with a swab stick, generally from the wall of the posterior fornix. In pregnant women who have only a slight discharge and extensive involvement of the vulva or labia, the specimens were collected from the irritated mucosa. The transport medium engaged was Amies to maintain viability and motility of trichomonads according to Dr.Van Dycke et al (1999). All the vaginal samples were collected voluntarily with the consent of the pregnant women and those who declined were omitted from this research.

Direct microscopy

All the samples were placed on a glass slide and depending on its fluidity; mix with a drop of physiological saline. Cover the direct preparation with a cover slip and examine microscopically at X400 magnification to detect yeast cells and presence of trichomonads. 10% Potassium hydroxide (KOH) was added to the preparation to increase the detection sensitivity of yeast cells, making the recognition of mycelia (pseudohyphae) much easier. Despite the fact that the sensitivity of wet mount is superior to that of a stained smear, all slides for this work were subjected to Gram Stain method of bacterial identification.

Gram staining techniques according to Monica Cheesbrough (2000) was applied.

Reagents used were;

Crystal violet stain

Lugol`s Iodine

Acetone- alcohol decolorizer

Safranine or neutral red

Systematic staining techniques

Fix the dried smear with methanol for 2 minutes.

Cover the fixed smear with crystal violet stain for 60 seconds.

Wash off the stain with clean water.

Cover the smear with Lugol`s iodine for 60 seconds.

Wash off the iodine with clean water.

Decolorize rapidly (few seconds) with acetone-alcohol solution and wash immediately with clean water.

Cover the smear with Safranine or neutral red stain (counterstain) for 2 minutes.

Wash off the stain with clean water, wipe the back of the slide with clean gauze, allow to air dry in draining rack.

Examine microscopically for gram positive yeast cells.

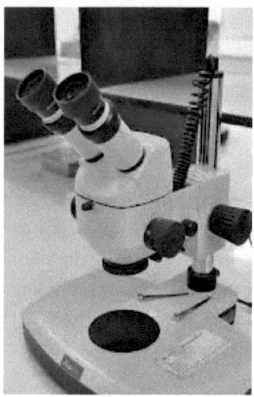

Figure A: Binocular Microscope in medical laboratory environment.

Figure B and C below, shows wet mount and gram stain of candida species in vaginal specimen.

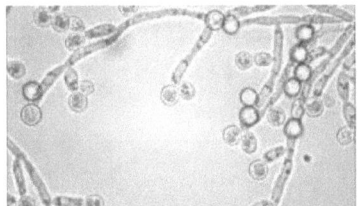

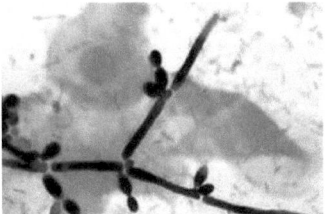

Figure B   Figure C

Figure D and E below, shows the jerky motility of trichomonas vaginalis suspended in wet mount preparation (D) and under stained condition (E) of high vaginal swab.

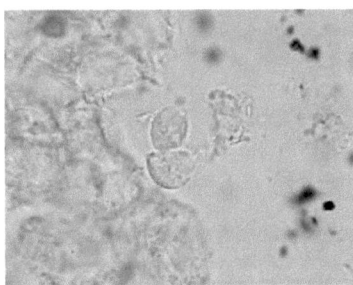

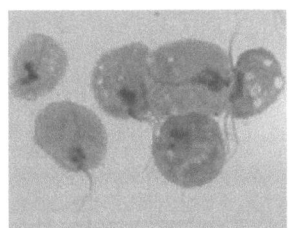

Figure D   Figure E

Results

Age group (years)	No. examined	No. infected	Frequency (%)
13-25	81	21	25.93
26-30	25	3	12.0
31-35	17	2	11.76
36-45	4	1	25.0
Total	127	27	21.26

Table 1: Age related frequency of Candida species infection from first of May to thirty-first July, 2013, research work, district of Porto Novo, Cape Verde.

Age group (Years)	No. examined	No. infected	Frequency (%)
15-25	81	6	7.41
26-30	25	1	4.0
31-35	17	1	5.82
36-45	4	0	0
Total	127	8	6.3

Table 2: Age related frequency of Trichomonas vaginalis infection from first of May to thirty-first July, 2013, research work, district of Porto Novo, Cape Verde.

Gravidity	Candida Species			Trichomoniasis vaginalis			Co-infection		
	N° examined	N° infected	Frequency (%)	N° examined	N° infected	Frequency (%)	N° examined	N° infected	Frequency (%)
Primigravidae	59	17	28.8	59	6	10.17	59	1	1.69
Multigravidae	68	10	14.71	68	2	2.94	68	0	0
Total	127	27	21.26	127	8	6.3	127	1	0.79

Table 3: Shows frequency distribution based on gravidity, from first of May to thirty-first July, 2013, research work, district of Porto Novo, Cape Verde.

Trimester	Candida Species			Trichomoniasis vaginalis			Co-infection		
First	N° examined	N° infected	Frequency (%)	N° examined	N° infected	Frequency (%)	N° examined	N° infected	Frequency (%)
0-12 weeks	31	5	16.13	31	1	3.23	31	0	0
Second 13-26 weeks	54	12	22.23	54	3	5.56	54	0	0
Third 27-40 weeks	42	10	23.81	42	4	9.52	42	1	2.38
Total	127	27	21.26	127	8	6.3	127	1	0.79

Table 4: Shows frequency of infection in relation to trimesters of pregnant women from first of May to thirty first July, 2013, research work, district of Porto Novo, Cape Verde.

Discussion

In this study, a total of one hundred and twenty seven pregnant women were subjected to research voluntarily, with age range of 13 to 45 years old. However, a total of 27 of the pregnant women were infected with candida species, making 21.26%, while 8 of the pregnant women were infected with trichomonas vaginalis, also making 6.3% of the population studied. The co-infection rate was 0.79% (infection of both candida species and trichomonas vaginalis). The infection of candida species among the pregnant population studied was mild and that of trichomonas vaginalis infection is low. It is important to observe that candida species infection is mostly a dominate infection than trichomonas vaginalis in this area of Cape Verde, the prevalence of candida species over trichomonas vaginalis is statistically significant, considering $P \leq 0.05$ for the method used.

The primigravidae recorded 59 (46.46%) and multigravidae recorded 68 (53.54%), the infection of candida species among primigravidae was 28.8% and 10.17% was reported in trichomonas vaginalis infection. The multigravidae infection of candida species was 14.71% and that of trichomonas vaginalis recorded 2.94%. However, the primigravidae was more infected with both candida species and trichomonas vaginalis than multigravidae.

The age distribution of 13 to 25 years old were more infected by candida species with 25.93%, while trichomonas vaginalis among this age group were slightly higher than other age groups of pregnant women amounting to 7.41% (see table 1 &2 above).

Trimesters of pregnant women also expressed slight changes with mothers in the third trimester (27 to 40 weeks) registered 23.81%, second trimester (13 to 26 weeks) was 22.23% and first trimester (0 to 12weeks) was 16.13% of candida species. The infection rate of trichomonas vaginalis recorded similar situation with third trimester 9.52%, second trimester 5.56% and first trimester 3.23%. The pregnant women in third trimester (27 to 40 weeks) were mostly attacked by these microorganisms of candida species and trichomonas vaginalis.

In relation to the general prevalence of the vaginal pathogens around the world, some researchers reported higher incidence whiles others were different. The prevalence rate of 21.26% recorded in this work corroborates with the findings of Drs. Klufio C A et al (1995) that reported 23 % of candida species infection among the pregnant people of papua, Simoes JA et al (1998) reported 19.2% in Brazilian pregnant women, and Lisiak M et al (2000) reported 20.8% of candida species in Polish pregnancy.

The infection of candida species has been dominating in juvenile pregnant women younger than or equal to 25 years old (25.93%), this also corroborates with the findings of Kent H (1991) and Bohbot JM (1995). This is also observed as regards to the infection of trichomonas vaginalis in this study. Although age may not necessarily be a serious factor that affects candidiasis prevalence, since all age groups studied were infected.

This is suggestive that, perhaps due to poor development of resistance to these infections among the very young, together, the Porto Novo data suggested a possible increase in vaginal immunity with age. The Porto Novo data also corroborates with research findings of Drs. Feyi-Waboso & Amadi (2001), which reported more candidiasis attack on primigravidae.

The prevalence of 21.26% of candidiasis infection recorded in Porto Novo, Cape Verde is higher than 14% prevalence study of candidiasis stated by Meda et al (1997) among Burkina Faso pregnant women, but it is interesting to observe here that age group up to 25 years old, represented the peak of childbearing in Porto Novo, Cape Verdean society, while pregnant women of age group up to 45 years were the least registered. This shows that this age group might be passing the childbearing age and approaching towards menopause, and if this age group is pregnant, they constitute a risk type of pregnancy. Nevertheless, as mentioned earlier in this work, advance in age, reduces the effect of oestrogen hormone in women, which in turn leads to decreased infective rate of candidiasis as women advances in age. The multigravidae groups of women have acquired knowledge and experience relating to pregnancy and its associated infections. They became better acquitted with information obtained through antenatal lectures, programs, and demonstrations, while the primigravidae were less experienced, hence, this could contribute to the high prevalence of candidiasis observed among them.

Conclusion

- Pregnant women are more vulnerable to vaginal candidiasis regardless of their age, trimester and parity, so treatment measures under the orientation of a nurse or general physician, should be implemented and infection will resolve in a short period of time.
- Avoidance of contributing factors, for example douching, wearing tight underwear and inadequate hygienic practice.
- Indiscriminate use of antibiotics without medical orientation should be discouraged.
- Education of pregnant women through seminars, campaign slogans and media transmission system, stressing the dangers of these infections and ways for prevention and control strategies.
- Further research is necessary for all wet mount or direct examination negative samples, using diagnostic sensitive and specific techniques.

References

Akinbiyi AA et al (2008): Prevalence of candida albicans and bacterial vaginosis in asymptomatic pregnant women in South Yorkshire, United Kingdom. Arch. Gynaecol Obstet 278: 463-466.

Aral SO et al (1992): Vaginal douching among women of reproductive age in the United States, 1988. Am J public health 82:210-14.

Bennett C (1993): The black population in the United States: march, 1992, current population reports. Washington: US bureau of census: 1993. Pub. No. P20-471 page 5.

Bohbot JM (1995): Les mycoses ganitales chroniques. Physiopathologie, traitement: Jusqu ou aller? Realites en gynecologic- obstetrique 5:29- 38.

British Association for sexual health and HIV (2007): Management of vulvovaginal candidiasis.

Cates W Jr. (1999): Estimates of the incidence and prevalence of sexually transmitted disease in the United States: American social health Association panel. Sex Transm Dis 26(4) suppl: S2-7.

Centers for disease control and prevention: Division of STD prevention at www.cdc.gov/std.

Clinical knowledge summaries (2007): Candida- female genital.

Das- Neves J et al (2008): Local treatment of vulvovaginal candidiosis: general and practical considerations. Drugs 68(13): 1787.

Donders G G et al (2002): Impaired tolerance for glucose in women with recurrent vaginal candidiasis. Am J Obstet Gynecol 187(4): 989

Draper D et al (1998). Cystein proteases of trichomonas vaginalis degrade secretory leucocyte protease inhibitor. J infec Dis 178:815-9.

Eschenbach DA (2004): Chronic Vulvovaginal Candidiasis. New Eng J Med 351: 851-852.

Falagas ME et al (2006): Probiotics for prevention of recurrent vulvovaginal Candidiasis: a review: J Antimicrob Chemther. 58(2): 266-272.

Ferrer J (2000): Vaginal candidosis: epidemiological and etiological factors. Int. J Gynaecol Obstet 71 (suppl-1): S21-7.

Feyi- Waboso P A and Amadi AN (2001): The prevalence and pattern of vaginal Candidiasis in pregnancy in ABA. J of Medical investigation and practice vol 2:25-27.

Fidel PL (2005): Immunity in vaginal Candidiasis. Current Opin. Infect. Dis 18(2):107-111.

Garcia HM et al (2006): Prevalence of vaginal Candidiasis in pregnant women, identification of yeast and susceptibility to antifungal agent. Rev. Appl. Microbiol 30(1): 9-12.

Ghys PD et al (1995): genital ulcers associated with human immunodeficiency virus- related immunosuppression in female sex workers in Abidjan, Ivory Coast. J infec Dis 172:1371-4.

Hobbs MM et al (1999): Trichomonas vaginalis as a cause of urethritis in Malawian men. Sex transm dis 26:381-7

http://www.clinical-laboratory.blogspot.com/2013/067women-have-natural-bacterial-defense.

http://www.google.cv/imgres? What-laboratory-test-would-you-collect-to-identify-trichomonas-vaginalis.

http://www.mundoeducaçâo.com.br/doenças/candidaou-candidiase.

Kazmierczak W et al (2004): Frequency of vaginal infections in pregnant women in the department of perinatology and gynaecology in Zabrze. Ginekol Pol Dec. 75(12):932-6.

Kent H (1991): Epidemiology of vaginitis. Am J Obstet Gynecol 165:1168

Klufio CA et al (1995): Prevalence of vaginal infections with bacterial vaginosis, trichomonas vaginalis and candida albicans among pregnant women at the Port Moresby General Hospital antenatal Clinic. PNG Med J. 38 :163-171.

Klufio CA et al (1995): Prevalence of vaginal infections with bacterial vaginosis, trichomonas vaginalis and candida albicans among pregnant women at the Port Moresby General Hospital antenatal clinic. PNG Med J.09-38(3):163-71.

Kreiss J et al (1994): Association between cervical inflammation and cervical shedding of human immunodeficiency virus DNA. J infect Dis 170:1597-601.

Krieger JN (1981): Urologic aspects of trichomoniasis. Investigations in Urology 18:411-417.

Laga M et al (1993): Non- ulcerative sexually transmitted diseases as risk factors for HIV 1 transmission in women: result from a cohort study. AIDS 7:95-102.

Levin WC et al (1998): Increase in endocervical CD4 lymphocytes among women with non-ulcerative sexually transmitted diseases. J infect Dis 177: 167-74.

Limia OF (2004): Prevalence of candida albicans and trichomonas vaginalis in pregnancy. Gen. Med Obstet. Gynaecol & women Health 6:4

Lisiak M et al (2000): Vaginal candidiasis frequency of occurrence and risk factors. Ginekol Pol. 71:964-970.

Maleeha Aslam et al (2008): Vulvovaginal cadidiasis in pregnancy. Biomedica vol 24 Jan-Jun/BIO-C.

Monica Cheesbrough (2000): Laboratory identification of microorganisms. District laboratory practice in tropical countries Part 2. Pg38.

Nikolov A et al (2006): Vaginal candida infection in the third trimester of pregnancy. Akush Ginekol (sofia) 45 (6): 7- 9.

Njirjesy P (2008): Vulvovaginal Candidiasis and bacterial vaginosis. Infect Dis Clin North America 22(4): 637-652.

Nohmi T (1995): Suppression of anti-candida activity of murine neutriphils by progesterone in vitro: a possible mechanism in pregnant women's vulnerability to vaginal Candidiasis. Microbiol. Immune 39(6): 405-409.

Nwosu CO and Djieyep NA 2007): Candidiasis and trichomoniasis among pregnant women in a rural community in the semi-arid zone, north eastern Nigeria. West African J Med. 26 (1):17-9.

Octavio FL and Maria XL (2004): Prevalence of candida albicans and trichomonas vaginalis in pregnant women in Havana City by an immunologic latex agglutination test. Med Gen Med 6(4). 50.

Omar AA (2001): Gram stains versus culture in the diagnosis of vulvovaginal Candidiasis. East. Mediter Helath J 7(6): 925-934

Parveen N et al (2008): Frequency of vaginal Candidiasis in preganat women attending routine antenatal clinic. J Coll Physicians Surg Pak. 03-18 (3): 154-7.

Rughooputh S & Greenwell P (2005): Trichomonas vaginalis: Paradigm of a successful sexually transmitted organism. Br. J Biomed Sci. 62(4): 193-200.

Sardana S et al (1994): Epidemiologic analysis of trichomonas vaginalis infection in inflammatory smears. Acta Cytol 38:693-7.

Scholes D et al (1998): Vaginal douching as a risk factor for cervical Chlamydia trachomatis infection. Obstet Gynecol 91: 993-997.

Shira CS and Frank JS (2006): Viability of trichomonas vaginalis in urine: epidemiologic and clinical implications. Journal of clinical implications & Microbiology 44:3787-3789.

Simoes JA et al (1998): Prevalence of Cervicovaginal infections during gestation and accuracy of clinical diagnosis. Infect Dis Obstet Gynecol, 6:122-133.

Sutton M et al (2007). The prevalence of trichomonas vaginalis infection among reproductive age women in the United States, 2001 to 2004. Clinical infect Dis 45(10): 1319-26.

Ter Muelen J et al (1992): Risk factors for HIV infection in gynaecological in patients in Dar Es Salaam, Tanzania, 1988-1990. East Afr Med J 69: 688-92.

Uneke CJ et al (2006): Trichomonas vaginalis infections among pregnant women in South Eastern Nigeria: the public health significance. The internet journal of Gynaecology and Obtetrics 6(1):17-21.

Van Dyck et al (1999): Laboratory diagnosis of sexually transmitted diseases. WHO geneva. Pg 70 -74.

Watson M C et al (2001): Oral versus intra Cochrane database syst Rev. (4): CD002845.

World Health Organization,WHO (2001): <u>Global prevalence and incidence of selected curable sexually transmitted infections.</u>

Xu D J and Sobel JD (2004): <u>Candida vulvovaginitis in pregnancy, Division of infectious diseases.</u> Curr. Infect. Dis Ref. 6:56-59.

Young GL & Jewell D (2001): <u>Topical treatment for vaginal candidiasis in pregnancy.</u> Cochrane database syst Rev. (4): CD000225.

Appendix

Management of trichomonas infection

An antibiotic medicine called metronidazole is the common treatment.

- Metronidazole 400mg twice daily for 5 to 7 days is sufficient.
- Take the tablets after meals.
- A metallic taste is a common side effect.
- Do not drink alcohol while taking metronidazole.
- Do not take metronidazole during the first trimester of pregnancy; it can have adverse effects on the fetus.
- Metronidazole can get into breast milk, so during breast feeding, the standard 7 days treatment can be lowered so that the baby does not get a large dose or to limit the exposure of the baby to the drug.
- Tinidazole is an alternative antibiotic treatment for trichomonas infection.
- Sexual partners must be invited to receive treatment at the same time.
- Always consult your medical doctor, pharmacist or other healthcare professional to ascertain your treatment and repeat laboratory diagnosis for confirmation of total cure.

Management of candidiasis

Since all topical and oral azole therapies give a clinical and mycological cure rate of over 80% in uncomplicated acute vulvovaginal candidiasis, choice is a matter of personal preference, availability and affordability, (British Association for sexual health and HIV, 2007)

- Single Episode
- Topical azole, for example, Clotrimazole, miconazole. These are less expensive than their oral counterparts, but have some disadvantages.
- Oral triazole, for example, fluconazole or itraconazole.
- Single high dose oral triazole is effective as treatment for 3 to 7 days.
- Topical treatment may worsen burning symptoms in the first few days and the person may prefer oral treatment, if there is inflamed /oedematous vulva, Watson M C et al (2001).
- When there seems to be treatment failure, use a longer course, may be combining oral and topical treatment. Where azole has failed, it could be due to infection by candida glabrata and nystatin can be more effective option.
- 10% of women have mixed infection with bacteria, therefore send vaginal swab for culture and sensitivity testing.
- If recurrent infections of four or more episodes per year, send swabs for culture and sensitivity testing and exclude alternative diagnosis and underlying cause, Donders G G et al (2002).
- An induction period of 1 to 2 weeks with at least one week oral agent or 1 to 2 weeks of topical antifungal agent.

- This could be followed by a maintenance period of 6 months with oral fluconazole 100mg weekly or topical Clotrimazole 500mg weekly.
- Treatment can be stopped after 6 months and if recurrent infection returns, then repeat induction / maintenance therapy.
- Approximately 90% of women will remain disease free at 6 months and 40% at one year, (British Association for sexual health and HIV,2007)
- If infection occurs during the maintenance period, refer patients to consultant Mycologist, as it may be due to azole resistance.
- Non- albicans infection is harder to treat due to increased azole resistance, in these cases, nystatin, boric acid, or flucytosine may be used but under the supervision of a health care professional.
- There is absolutely no evidence to support the treatment of asymptomatic male sexual partners in either episodic or recurrent vulvovaginal candidiasis.

Candidiasis management in pregnancy

Young & Jewell (2001), recommended, longer courses of topical Clotrimazole, miconazole, econazole, and nystatin are less effective. Oral fluconazole and itraconazole must not be used during pregnancy or breast- feeding. If immunocompromised, especially HIV infection or diabetes, extend the treatment period to 7 to 14 days (British Association for sexual health and HIV, 2007).

Complications and prognosis

- Cure rate is 80% for uncomplicated cases.
- About 20% will have treatment failure; defined as persisting symptoms at 7 to 14 days (clinical knowledge summaries, 2007)
- Recurrent candidiasis; defined as more than four episodes per year, can affect up to 50 % of sufferers at a given period in their life time.
- Depression and psychosexual problems can occur in women who suffer recurrent episodes.
- Treatment during pregnancy is likely to relapse.

However, medical advice is needed in the following category of patients who have episodes of candidiasis:

- ✓ Age less than 16 or older than 60 years.
- ✓ Pregnant or breast feeding.
- ✓ Symptoms differing from normal, for example, malodorous discharge, ulcers, blisters.
- ✓ Two episodes in six months.
- ✓ Has had a previous sexual transmitted disease.
- ✓ Abnormal menstrual bleeding / lower abdominal pain.
- ✓ Adverse reaction to antifungal treatment or they are ineffective.
- ✓ Symptoms persist more than seven days.

Preparation of laboratory reagents used in this project study

Crystal violet Gram stain

Crystal violet 20g

Ammonium oxalate....9g

Absolute ethanol......1litre

- Weigh the crystal violet on a piece of clean paper. Transfer to a clean brown bottle already premarked to hold 1 litre.
- Add the absolute ethanol and mix until the crystal violet dye is completely dissolved. Prepare reagents away from an open flame.
- Weigh the ammonium oxalate and dissolve in about 200ml of distilled water. Add it to the stain and make it up to the 1 litre mark with distilled water, and mix well.
- Remember that ammonium oxalate is a toxic chemical, please handle with caution.
- Label the bottle, and store at room temperature. The stain is stable for several months.

Lugol's Iodine Solution

Potassium iodide.......20g

Iodine...................10g

Distilled water.........1 litre

- Weigh the potassium iodide, and transfer to a clean brown bottle premarked to hold 1 litre.
- Add little water and mix until the potassium iodide is completely dissolved.
- Weigh the iodine and add to the solution above and mix until the iodine is completely dissolved.
- Remember that iodine is injurious to health if inhaled or allowed to come in contact with the eyes, therefore handle with care in a well ventilated room.
- Make up to 1 litre mark with distilled water and mix well.
- Label the bottle, and mark it toxic. Store in a dark place at room temperature. Renew the solution if its color fades.

Acetone & alcohol decolorizer

Acetone.............500ml

Absolute ethanol...475ml

Distilled water......25ml

- Mix the distilled water with the absolute ethanol or methanol.
- Remember that ethanol and methanol are highly flammable; therefore keep away from an open flame.
- Measure the acetone and add to the alcohol solution and mix well.

- Remember also that acetone is highly flammable, chemical that vaporizes quickly; therefore use away from an open flame.
- Label the bottle, and mark it highly flammable, store in a safe place at room temperature. It is stable indefinitely.

Neutral red 0.1% w/v

Neutral red.......1g

Distilled...........1litre

- Weigh the neutral red on a piece of clean paper and transfer to a bottle of 1 litre capacity.
- Add little water and mix until the dye is fully dissolved.
- Make up to 1 litre mark and mix well.
- Label the bottle and store at room temperature. The stain is stable for several months.

Hospital do Porto Novo

Laboratorio Analises Clinicas

Pesquisa sobre saude de mulheres gravida em Porto Novo

Por favor estamos a realizar um trabalho de pesquisa sobre saude de mulheres gravida em Porto Novo, para um period de 3 meses (Maio , Junho e Julho, 2013). Gostaria de faze-la?

Se quiser, entâo fazemos.

Numero----------------------------

No	Idade	Parity	Trimester	Candida spp	Trichomonas Vaginalis	Co-infection